take a peek:

Inside this book, you´ll find a variety of designs to get your hands on and start coloring

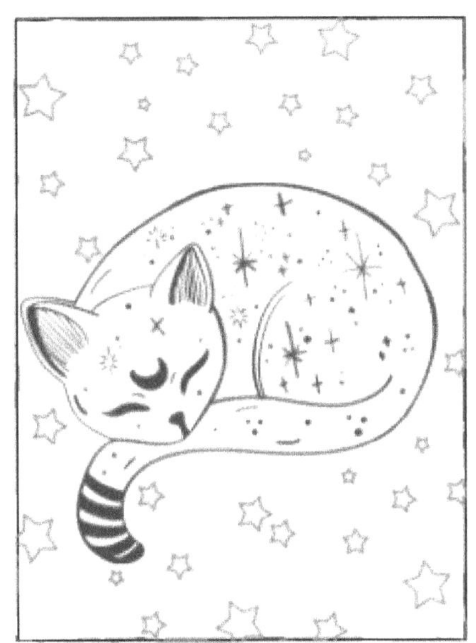

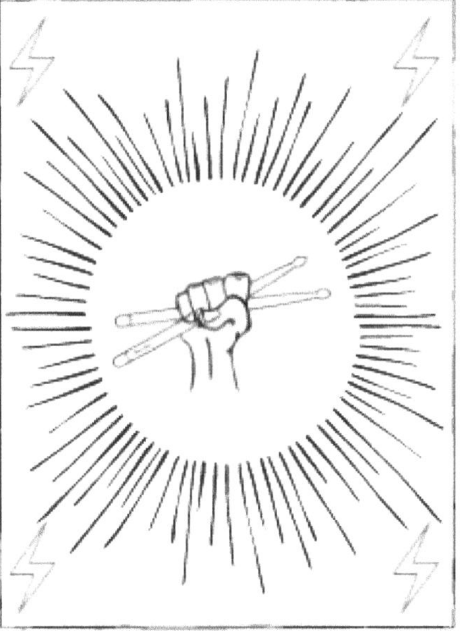

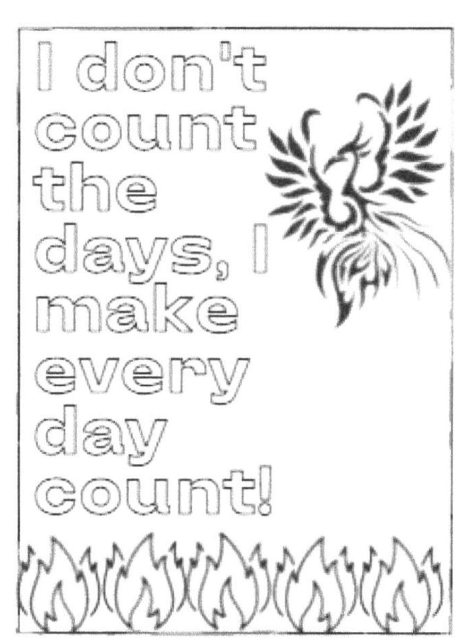

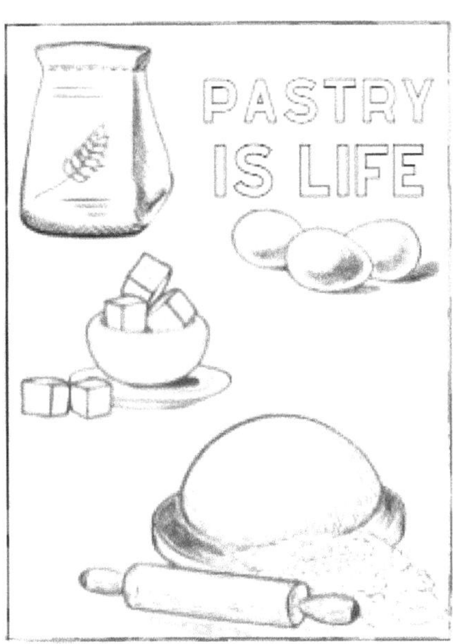

This book's very own heart and soul is to help you, our final recipient, overcome the difficult situation you are facing. It´s with our hopeful thoughts that we expect you to have a creative distraction from the pain and/or hard time you are enduring. Behind every page, there´s a blank one with a gift label just in case you want to dedicate the colored image to someone you care about. Feel free to crop the page. Enjoy!

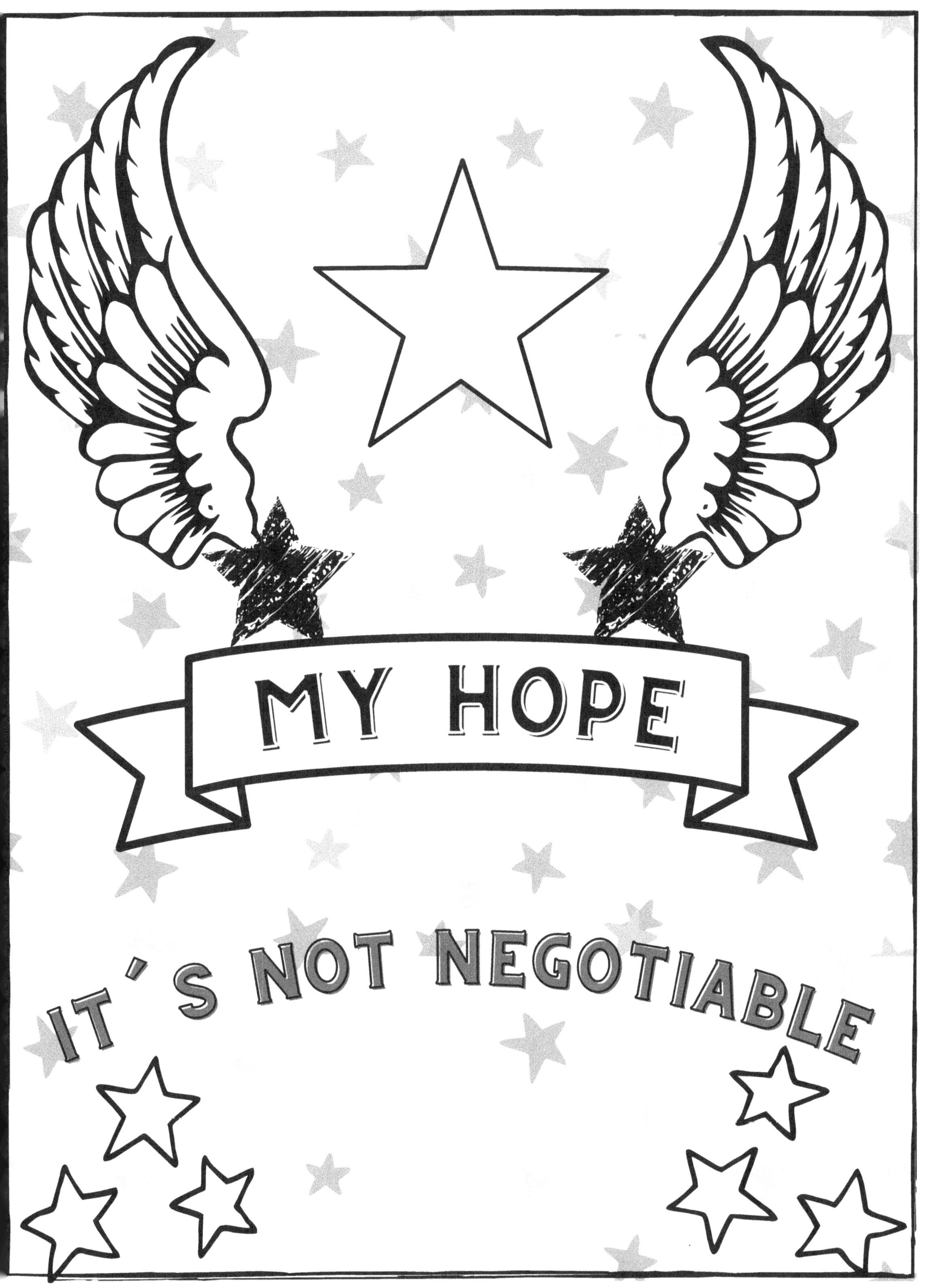
MY HOPE
IT´S NOT NEGOTIABLE

Completed on:____/____/_____

From:___________ To:_____________

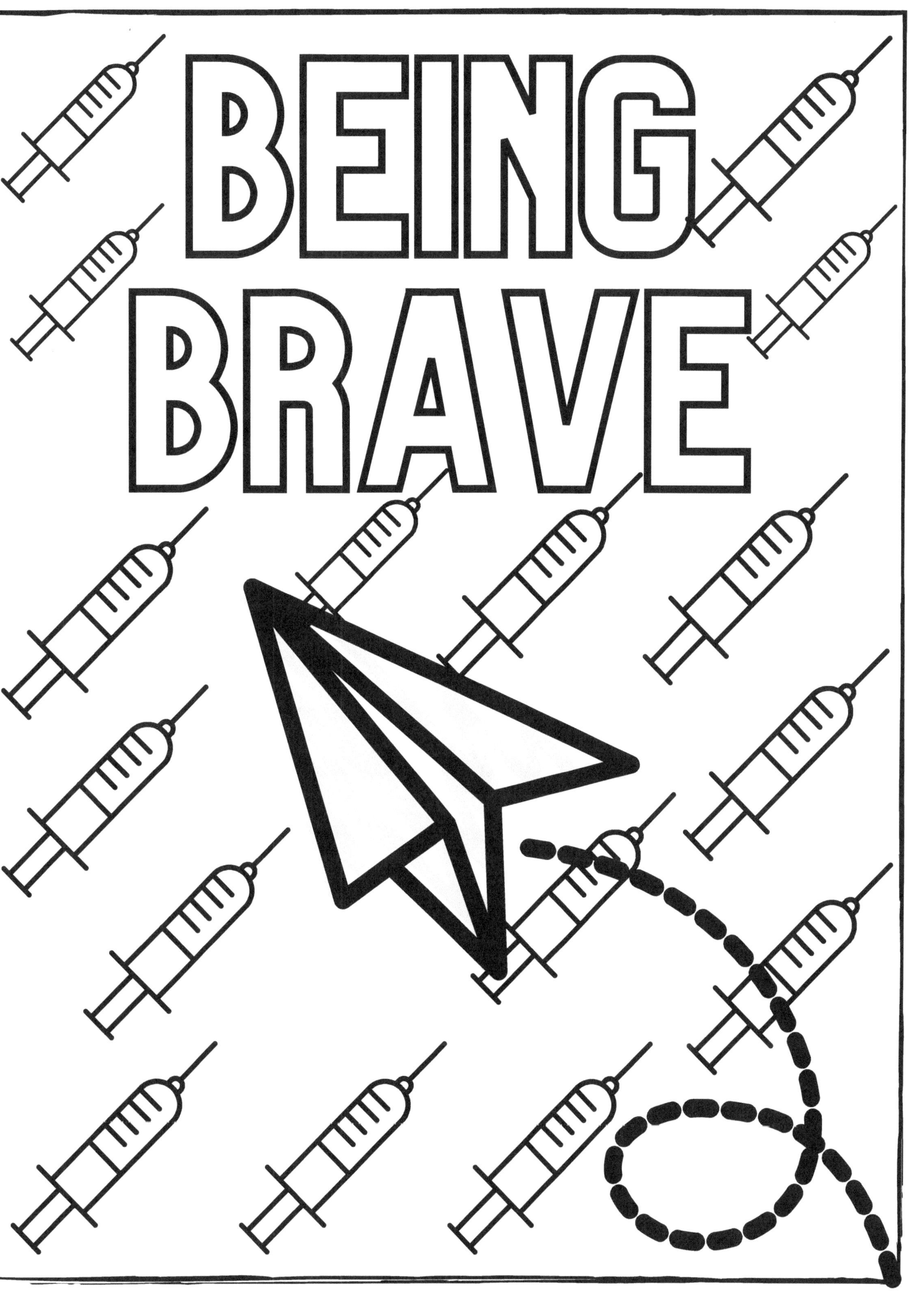
BEING
BRAVE

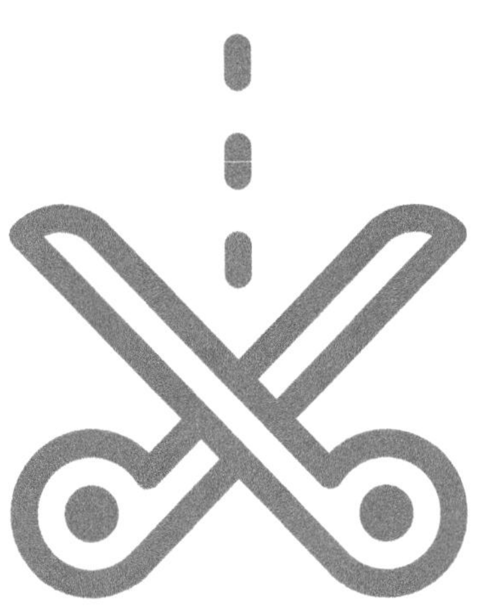

Completed on:____/____/_____

From:___________ To:_____________

Pain doesn´t define me... it refines me

Completed on:_____/_____/______

From:____________ To:_______________

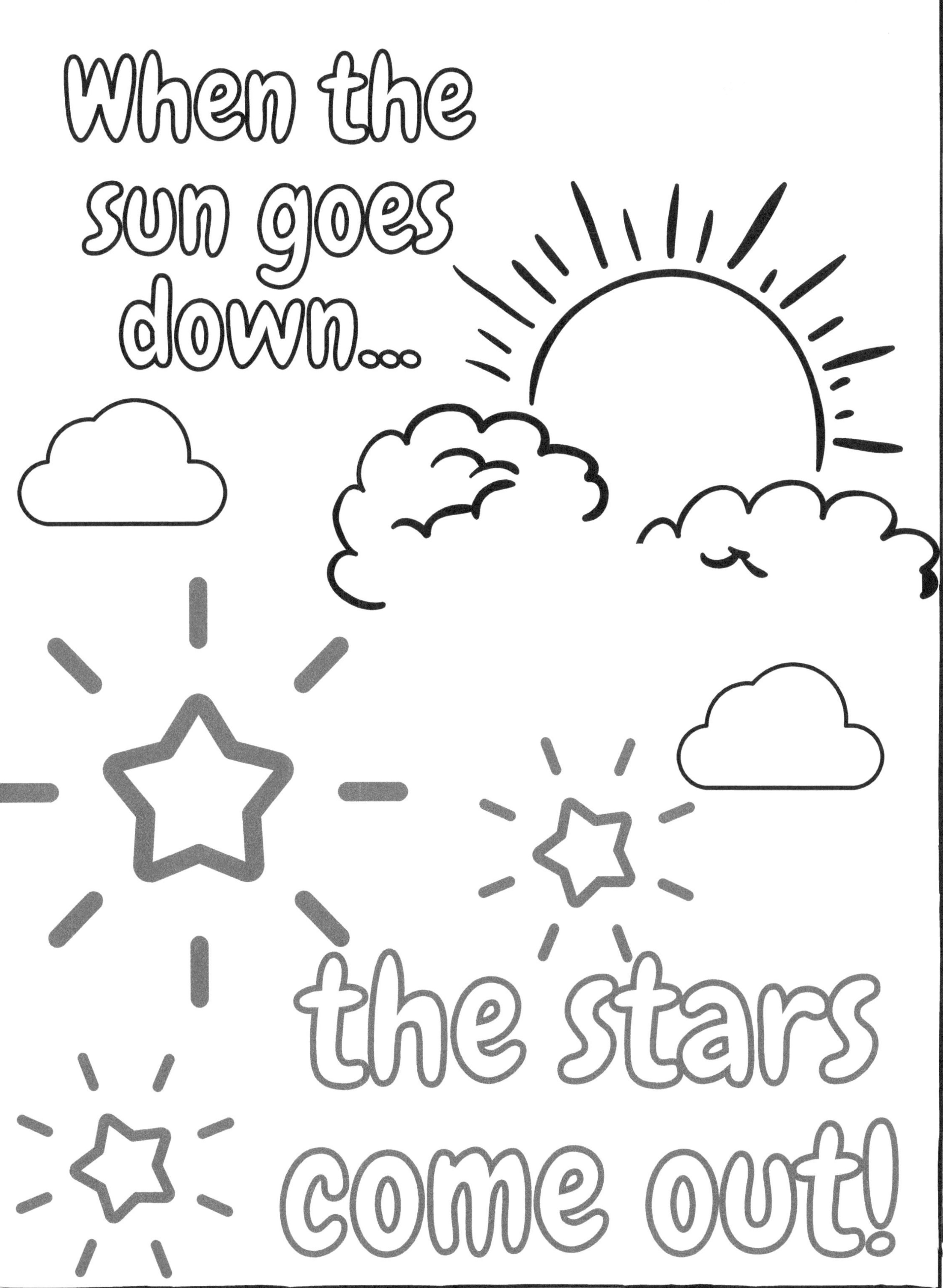
When the sun goes down...
the stars come out!

Completed on:____/____/_____

From:___________ To:_____________

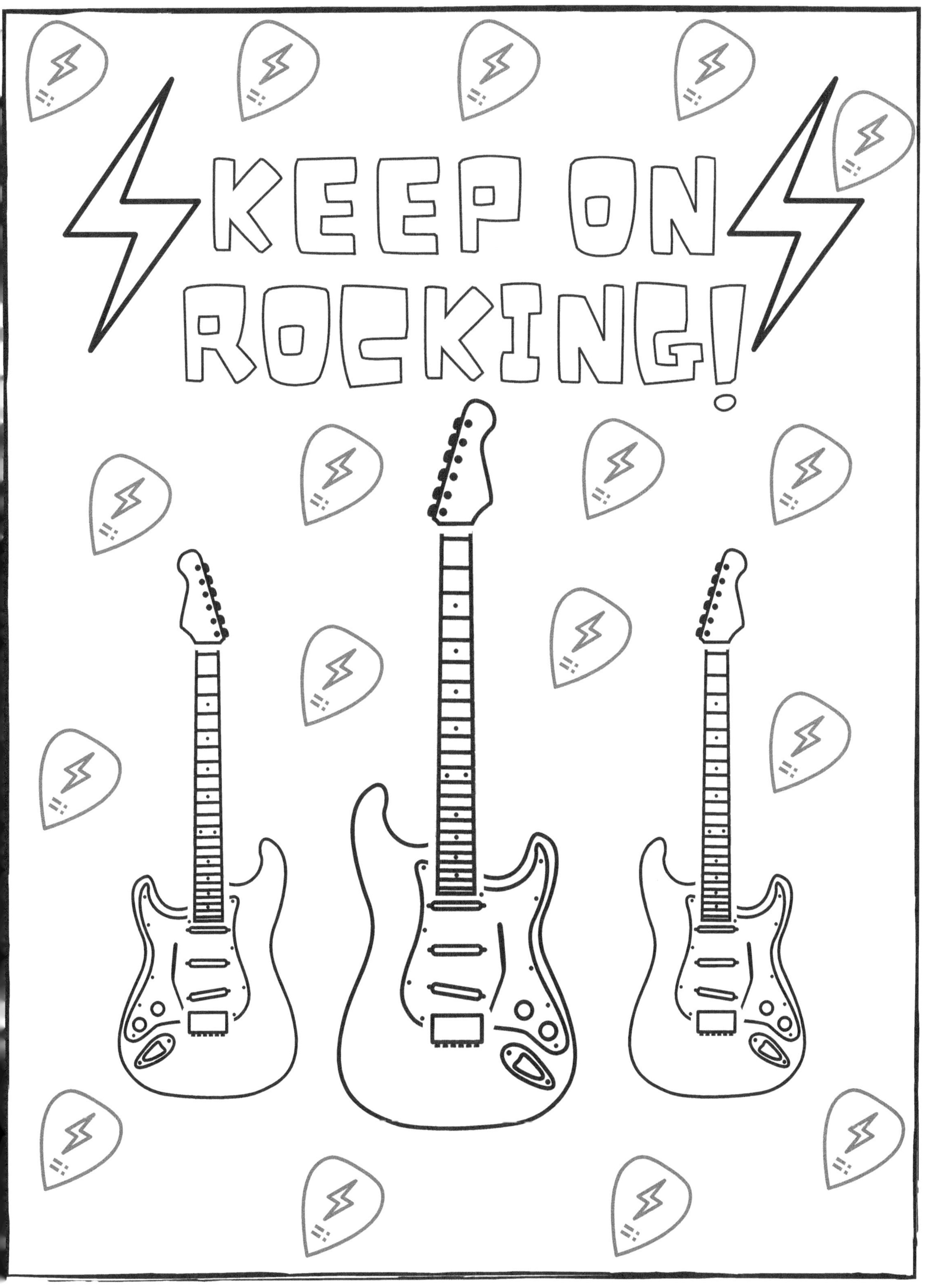
KEEP ON
ROCKING!

Completed on:_____/_____/______

From:_____________ To:________________

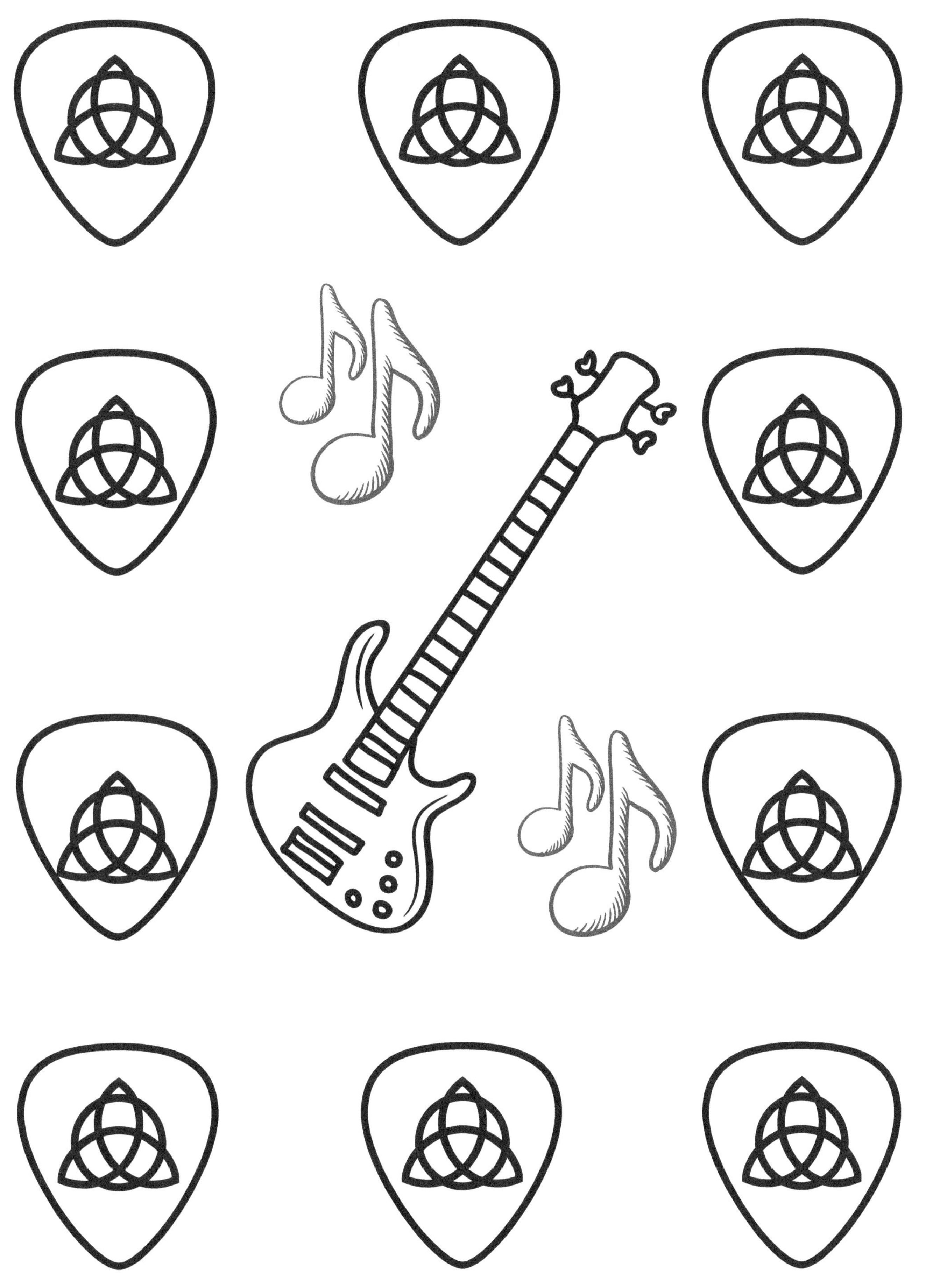

Completed on:____/____/_____

From:___________ To:_____________

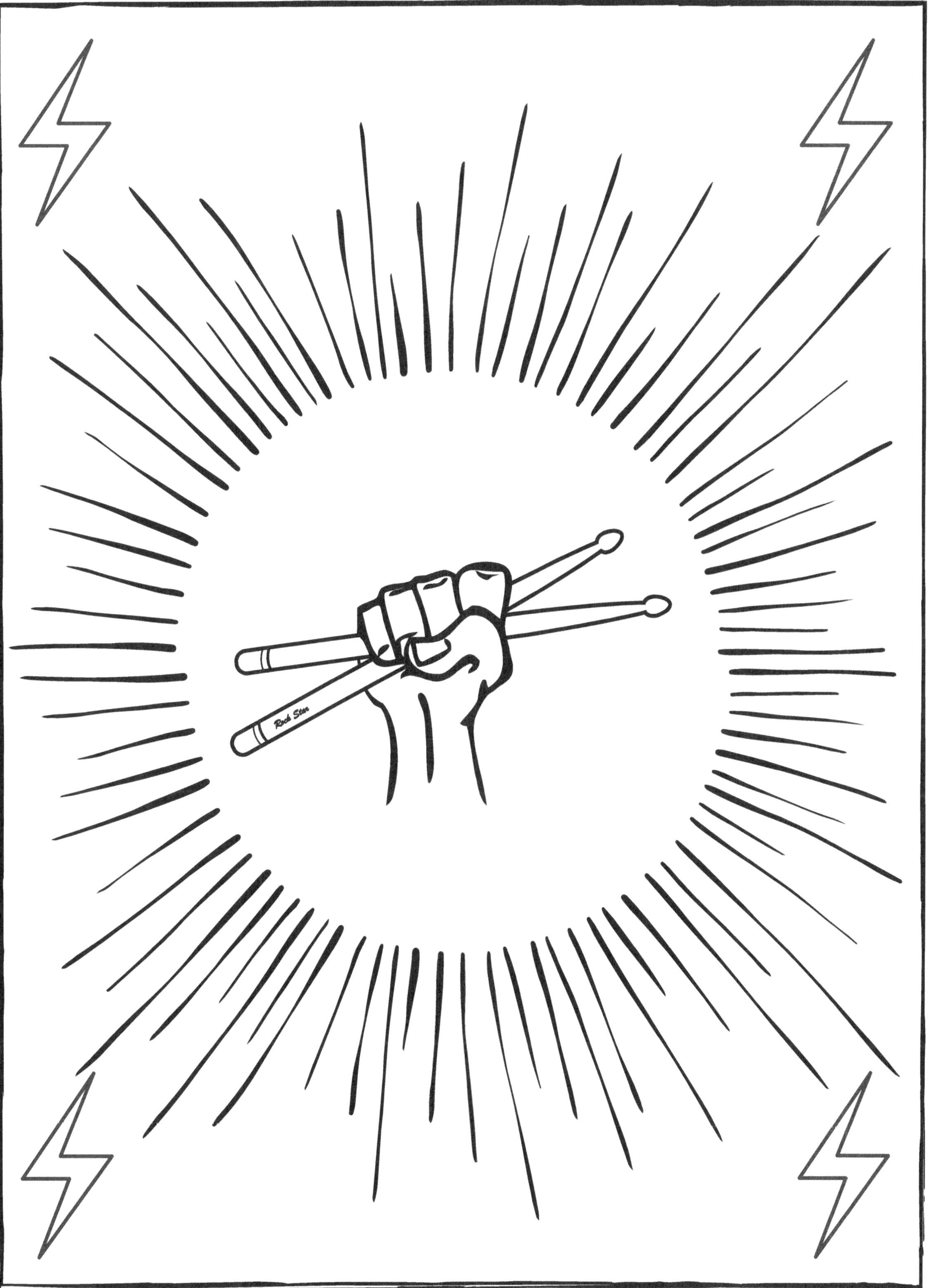
Rock Star

Completed on:_____/_____/______

From:_____________ To:________________

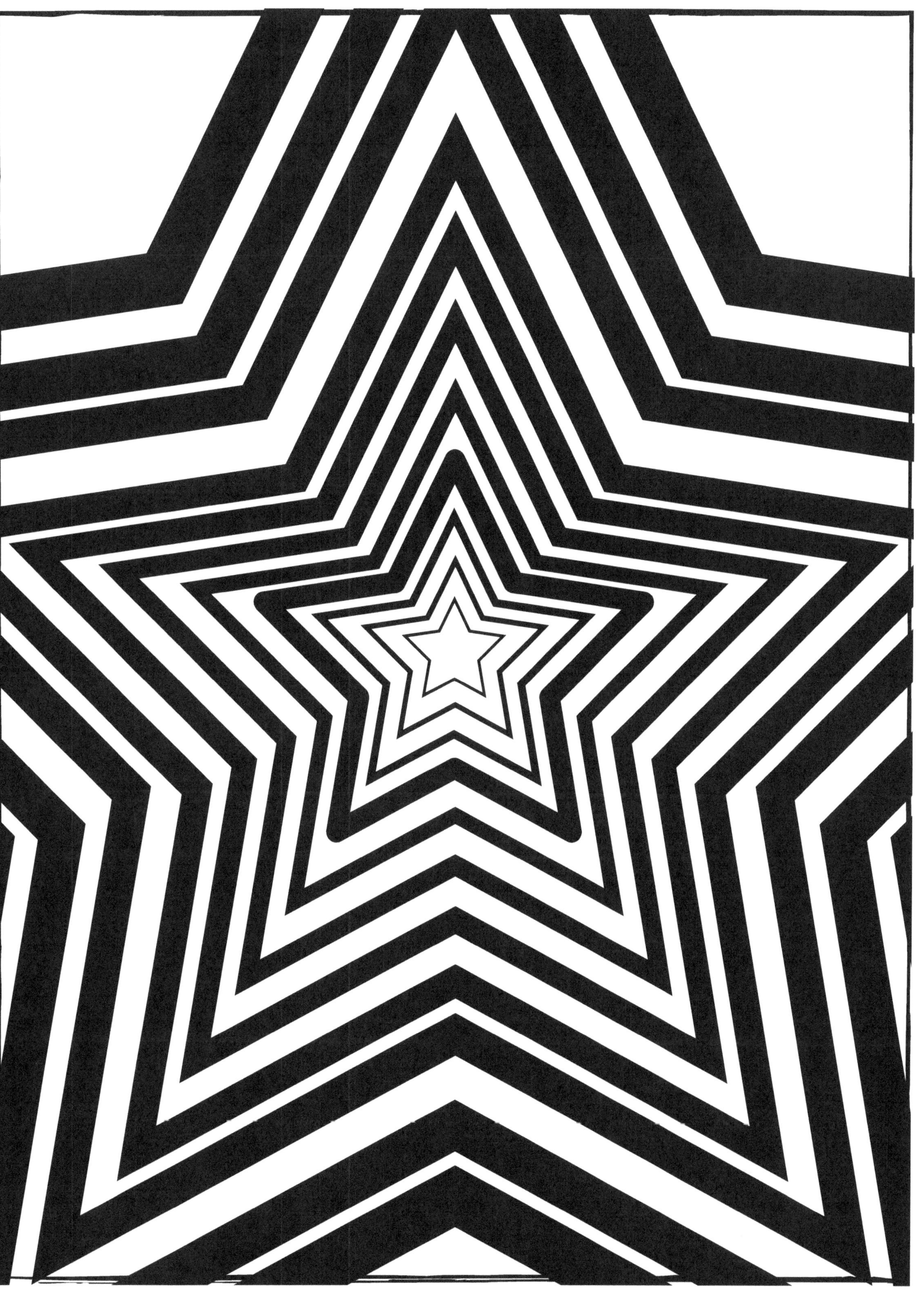

Completed on:____/____/_____

From:___________ To:_____________

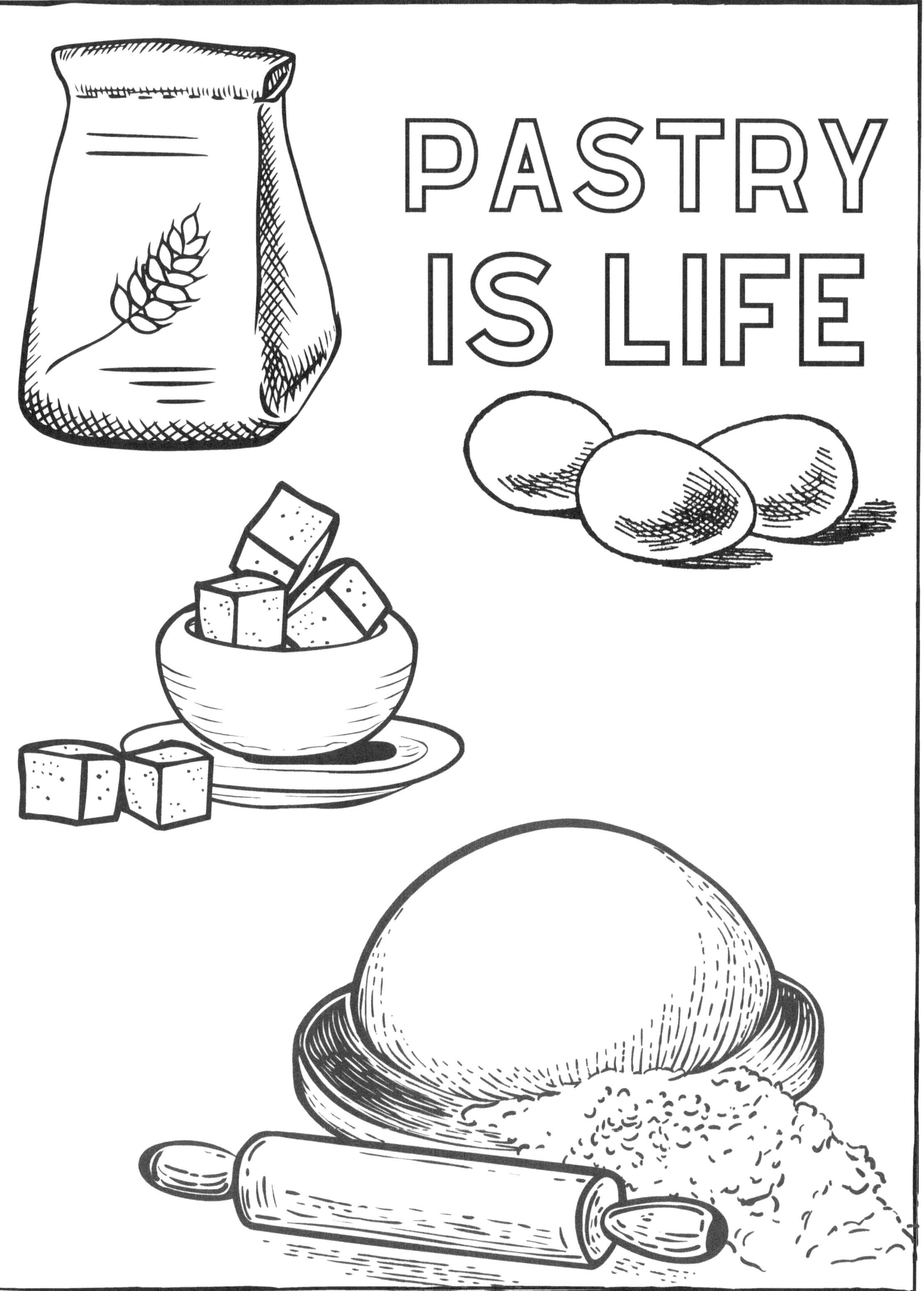
PASTRY
IS LIFE

Completed on:____/____/_____

From:___________ To:_____________

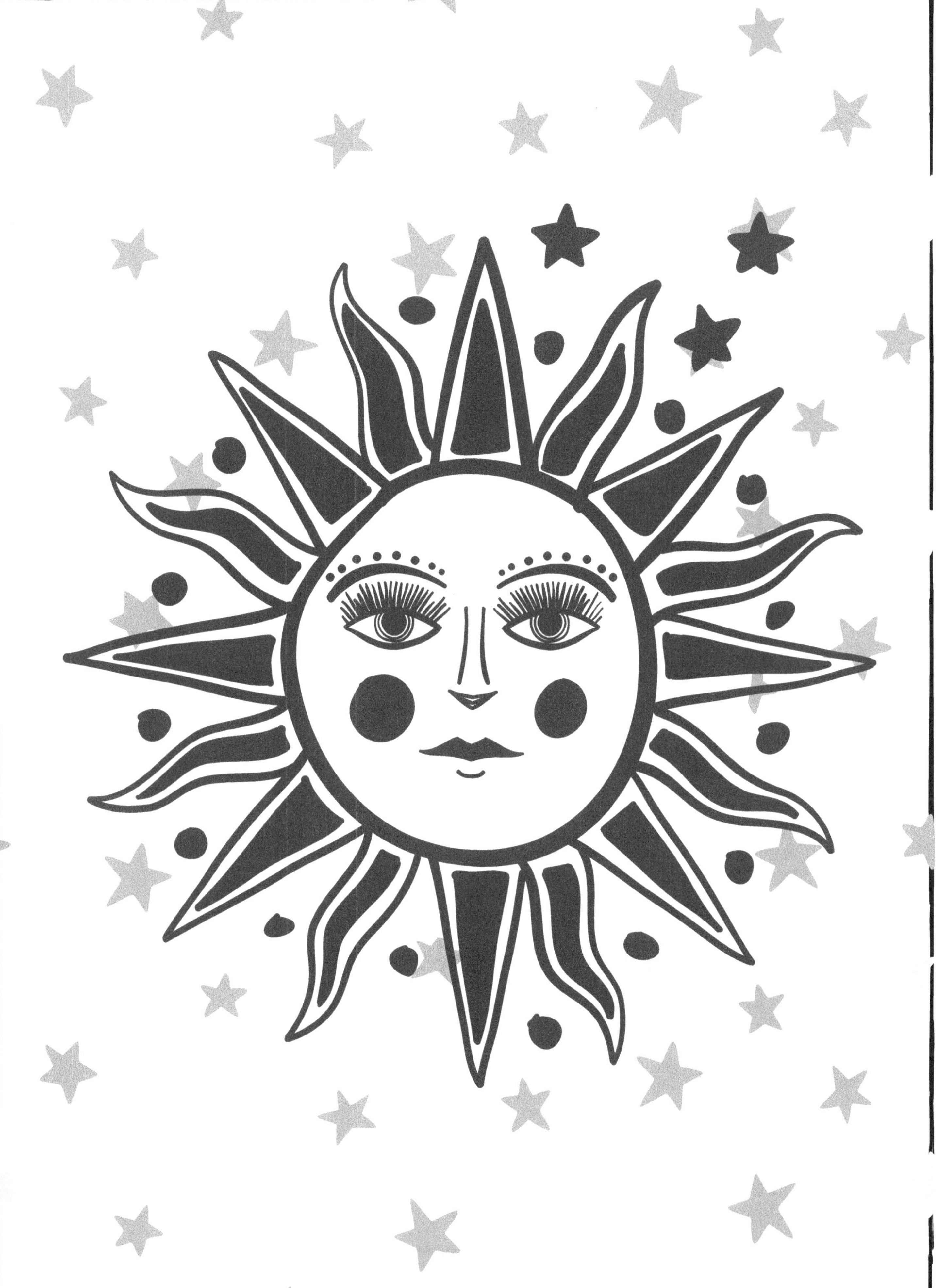

Completed on:_____/_____/______

From:_____________ To:_________________

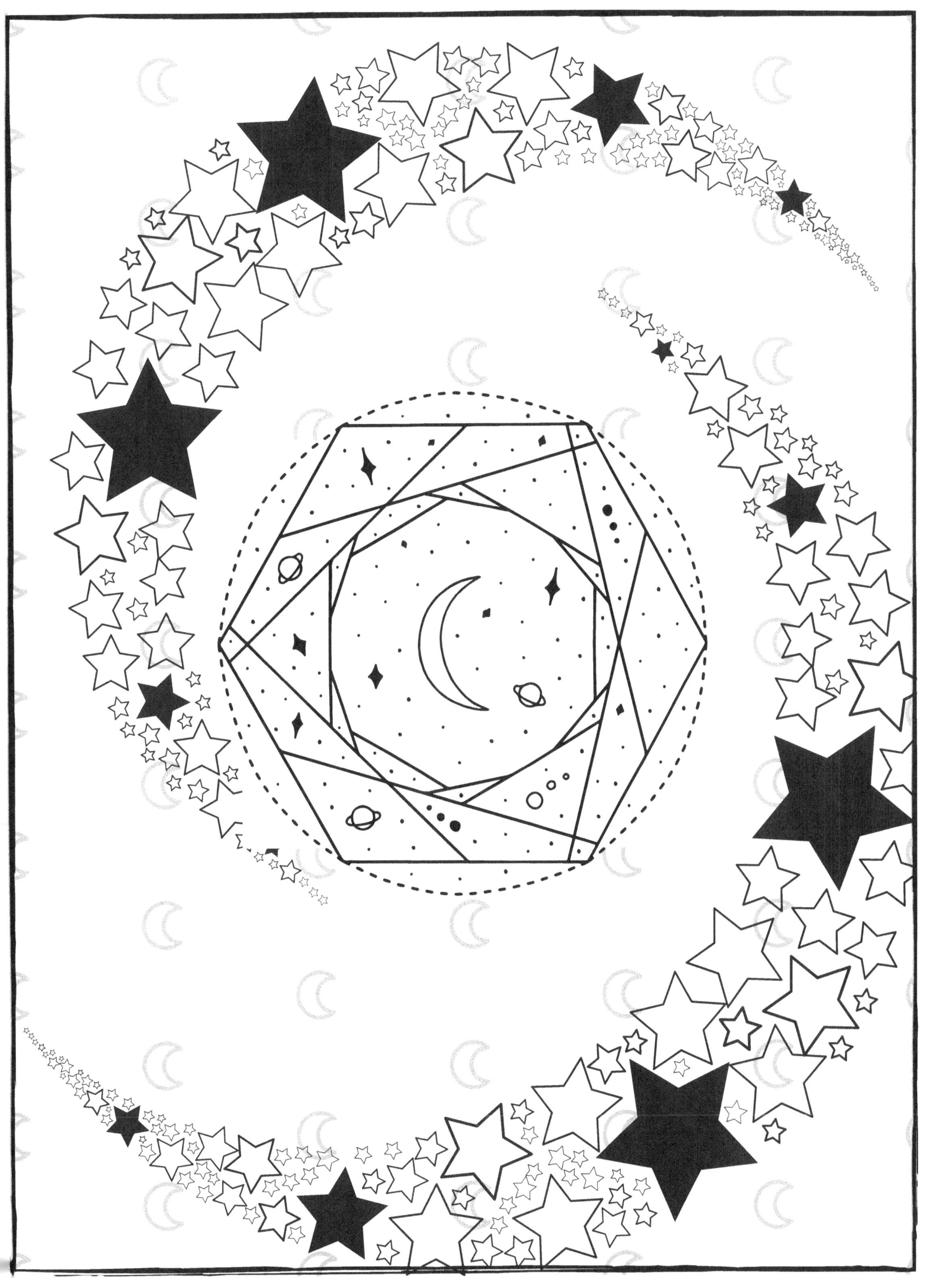

Completed on:____/____/_____

From:___________ To:______________

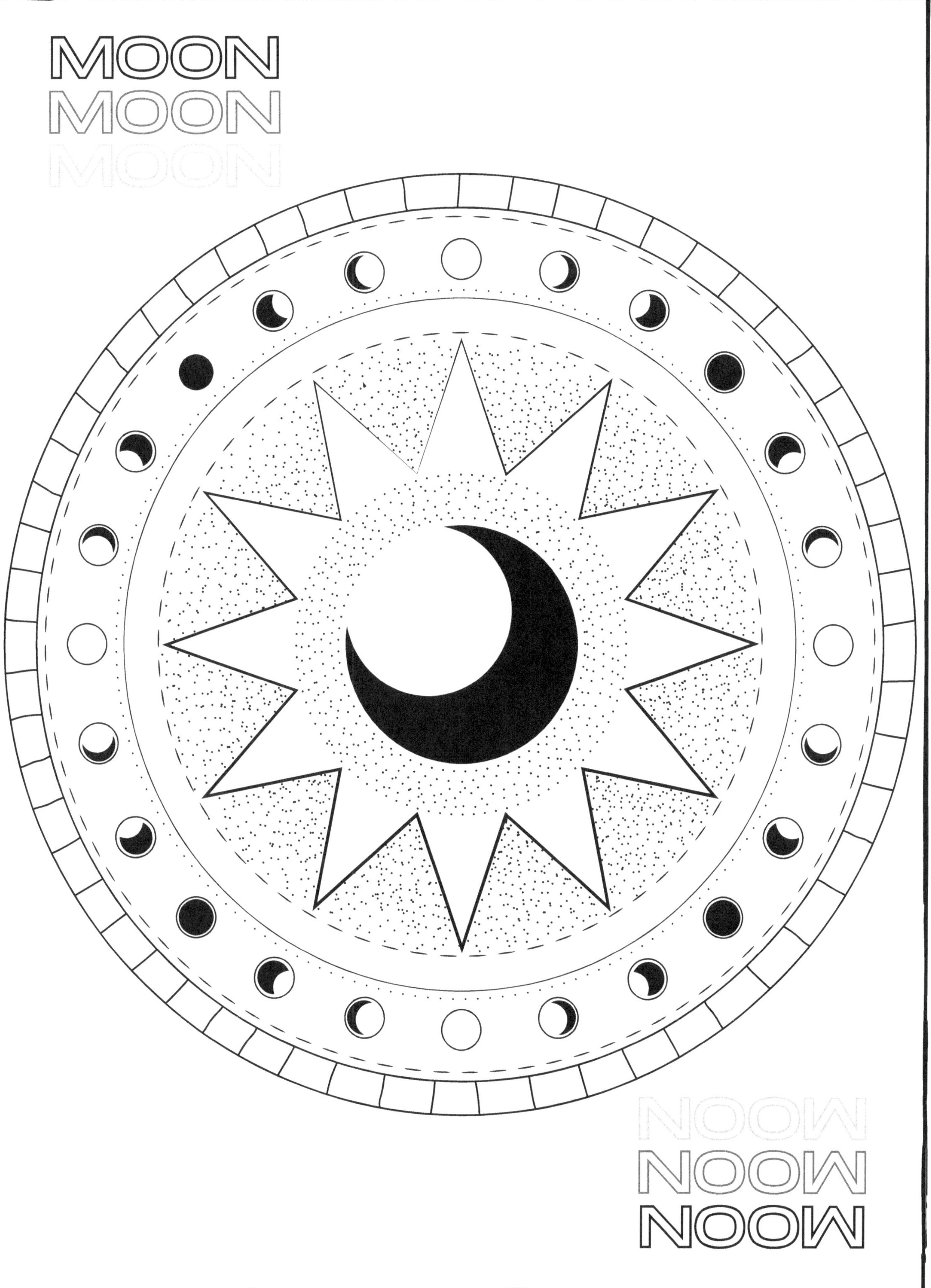
MOON
MOON
MOON
MOON
MOON
MOON

Completed on:____/____/_____

From:___________ To:_____________

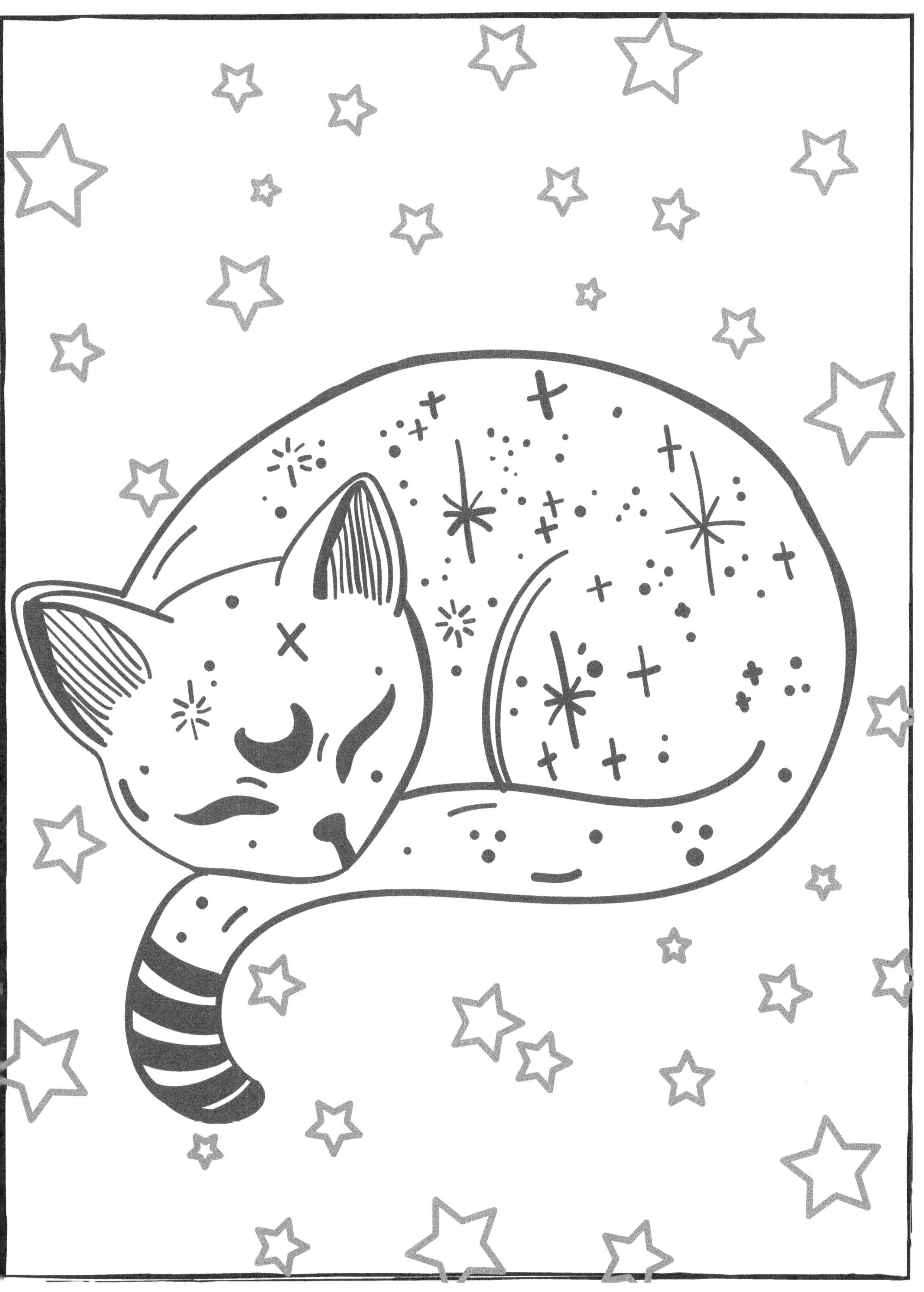

Completed on:____/____/_____

From:___________ To:_____________

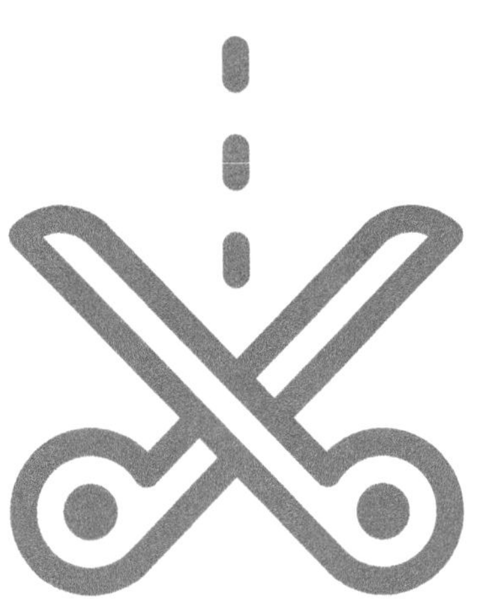

Completed on:____/____/_____

From:___________ To:_____________

One day at the time

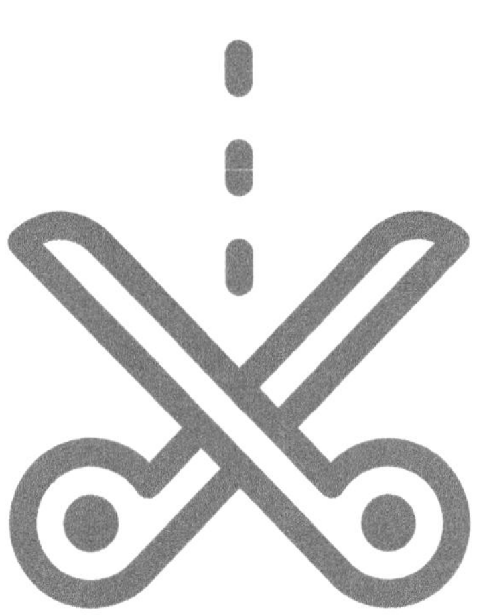

Completed on:____/____/_____

From:___________ To:______________

I WILL NOT GIVE UP!

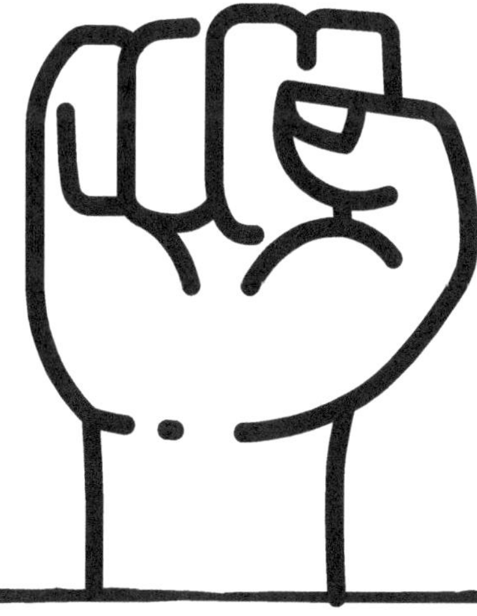

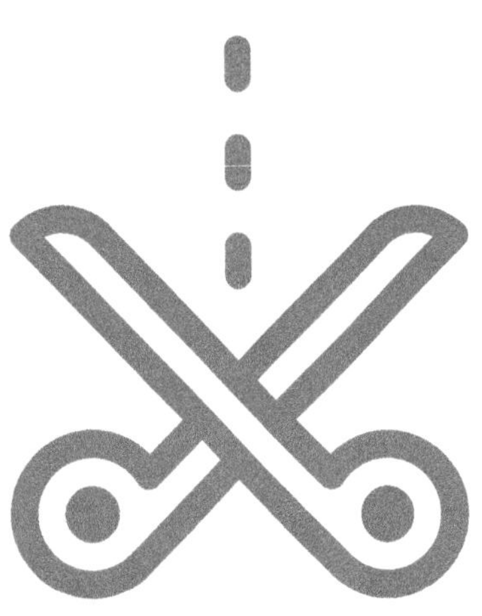

Completed on:____/____/_____

From:___________ To:_____________

I'M NOT ALONE IN THIS

Completed on:____/____/_____

From:___________ To:_____________

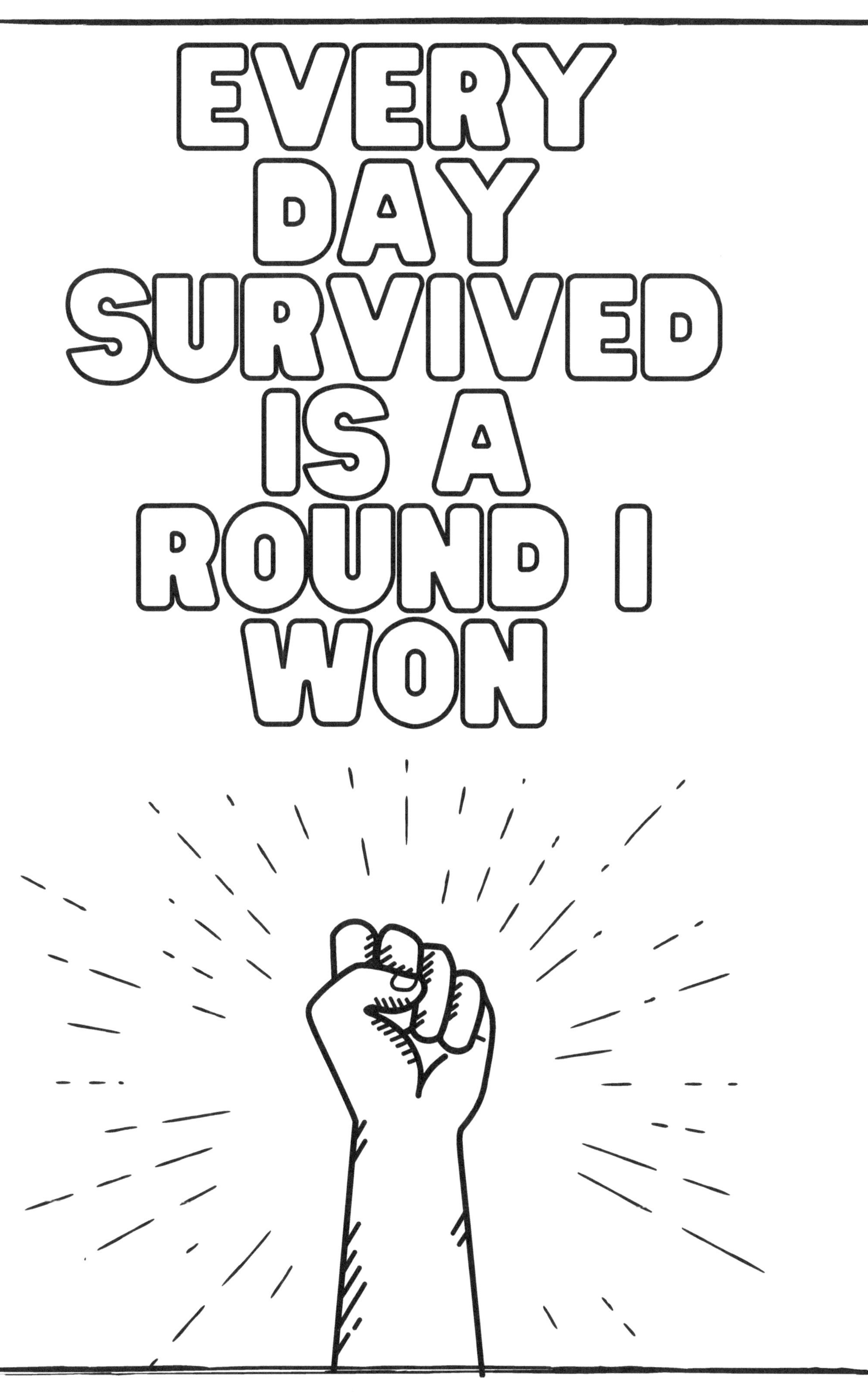
EVERY
DAY
SURVIVED
IS A
ROUND I
WON

Completed on:____/____/_____

From:___________ To:______________

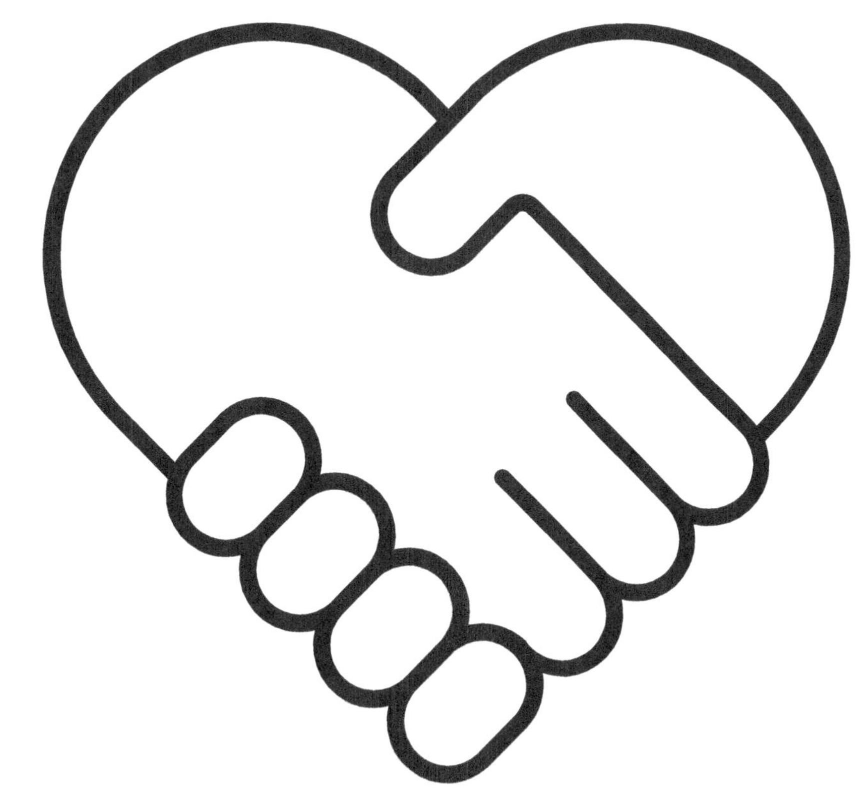

THANK YOU FOR BEING HERE

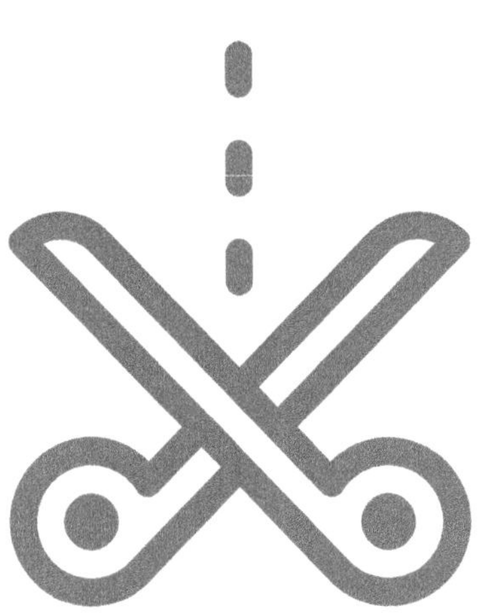

Completed on:____/____/_____

From:___________ To:_____________

I don't count the days, I make every day count!

Completed on:_____/_____/______

From:______________ To:________________

www.ingramcontent.com/pod-product-compliance
Lightning Source LLC
Chambersburg PA
CBHW081636250726
48657CB00009B/2903

* 9 7 9 8 5 2 8 0 5 8 7 3 3 *